Complete Chest Development
Revised Edition

Written and Published by Bill Pearl
Edited by George and Tuesday Coates
Layout and Illustrations by Richard R. Thornley Jr.

Copyright © 1963-2015 Bill Pearl

Bill Pearl
P.O. Box 1080
Phoenix, Oregon 97535
Email: support@billpearl.com
Website: www.billpearl.com

ISBN-13: 978-1-938855-09-2

Notice of Rights

All rights reserved. No part of this book may be reproduced or transmitted in any form by any means, electronic, mechanical, photocopying, recording, or otherwise, without the prior written permission of the publisher.

Medical Disclaimer - See Your Doctor

Most people may do all of the exercises found in this book with no ill effects. However, if certain movements cause discomfort they should be eliminated. See your doctor and get the doctor's approval on the total fitness program.

Table of Contents

Chapter 1

Introduction

Chest development is very important, not only from the stand point of health, but for one's general physical appearance. A large chest denotes health and vitality. One's physical strength is closely associated with a large, fully developed chest.

Pictures best describe the proper way to do exercises. Make use of them to eliminate errors.

All of you are aware of the part your lungs play in physical wellbeing. Do not neglect them; emphasize deep breathing when you exercise.

Our exercise illustrations and the programs we have outlined are designed to help you develop a better and larger chest

Good Luck!
Leo Stern

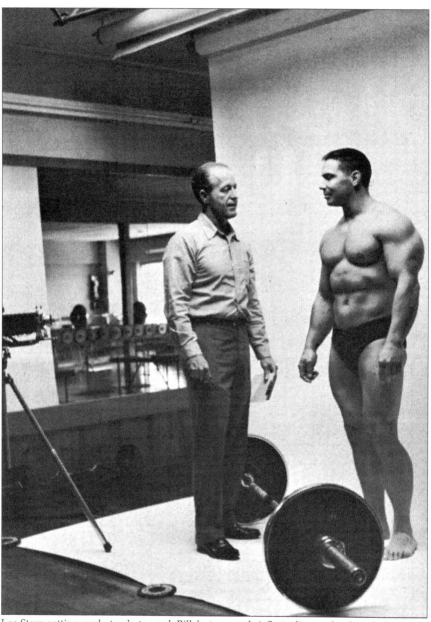

Leo Stern getting ready to photograph Bill, but pauses briefly to discuss the shoot before snapping the shutter.

Chapter 2

Complete Chest Development

A large thick chest that is muscled and has good depth is something that every true body builder should strive for. It should be realized how important it is to the general appearance of the upper body, but still how important it is to the general well-being of the person.

Well-toned muscles of the chest, help a person stand more erect, as well as keep the organs of the chest and stomach in their proper place. This is important to a person's health as a young man and the older a person gets, the more important it becomes. As for appearance, we know that a person with a large muscular chest is impressive. It has always been a symbol of health and manliness.

The reason for writing the Big Chest Book is not to build an impressive chest for vanity's sake, but to help a person train properly and help the advanced man think a little, if he is not doing justice to that area of the body.

I am not as fortunate as some to have a chest that is naturally thick or a large rib box expansion. This has always been an area of my body that has taken considerably more work and effort. Perhaps because of this I feel I am a little more of an authority on this than some others because of the hundreds of hours I have spent on myself to obtain what I now have. I have tried everything I have ever heard of for improving the chest and have invented several movements that have not been seen by myself before. What we have in this book are the best that I know. They are exercises that will work the muscles of the chest as well as emphasize the rib cage.

Let me emphasize the importance of doing all of the exercises as they are written and to be sure to do them as strictly as possible. Do not handle weight that is too heavy for you. Concentration while training is something that cannot be stressed enough.

Train hard and keep a positive attitude towards your workouts. With consistency, you are sure to make the improvements you are looking for.

Best of Luck,
Bill Pearl

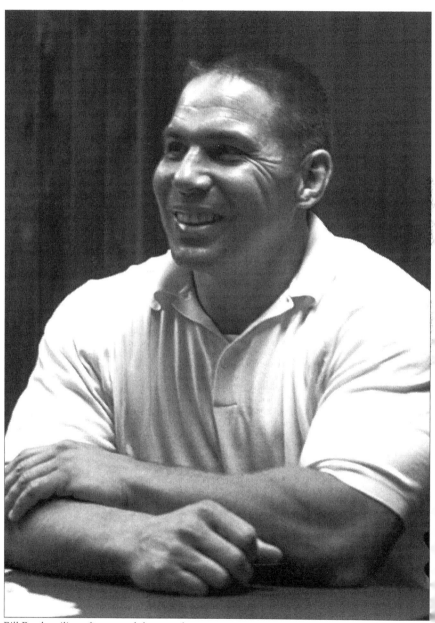

Bill Pearl smiling after a good days work.

Chapter 3

How to Use this Book

If a person is interested in weight training for more than basic conditioning, it is imperative that he study each illustration and description before attempting a new exercise. Progress definitely can be deterred if an exercise is done incorrectly.

Many exercises can be accomplished with the exact same motion but will affect different areas of a muscle by the angle at which the exercise is performed. For example: an exercise done on a flat bench, or an incline bench, will put different emphasis on the same muscle even though the same motion, weight and equipment are used.

It is therefore necessary to perform exercises from as many different angles that are reasonable and to use as many variations that are reasonable to develop a fully matured muscular physique.

On the following pages, highly accurate drawings appear that will enable you to see the pieces of equipment used to perform each exercise and the style used for each movement. Each exercise includes the proper name of the exercise, the muscle group most affected, "degree of difficulty" information, and a written description of how the exercise should be done.

The "degree of difficulty" information appearing below each exercise heading will give you at a glance what exercise may be suited for your present physical condition.

NOTE: It is not necessarily true that an exercise considered "easy" may not be just as effective as one considered "hard". Any exercise can be made more or less difficult, depending on the weight used or the effort put forth.

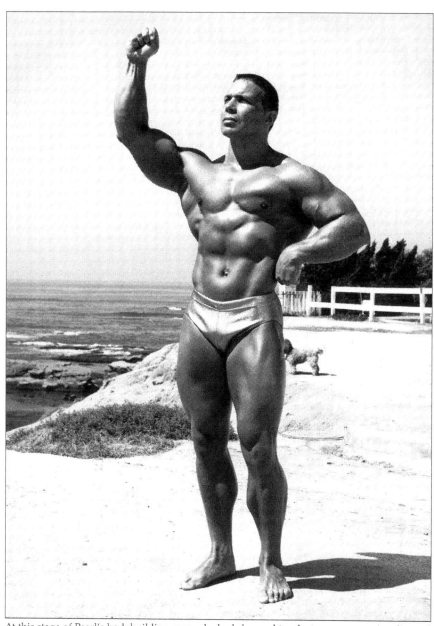

At this stage of Pearl's bodybuilding career, he had changed to a lacto-ovo-vegetarian diet and was still able to maintain his massive size throughout his entire body.

Chapter 4

Training Advice

Specialization

When specializing on the chest, start training program with a light warm-up exercise; next, do some abdominal exercises followed by leg work. A very fine exercise for enlarging the rib cage is breathing squats. A full description of this exercise will be found in our book, Building Bulk and Power. Immediately after doing breathing squats, do a set of either bent arm laterals or incline press. Use a light poundage so that full expansion and stretching of the chest can be accomplished. The barbell pullover or the dumbbell pullover can also be used.

When doing heavy squats, use a chest exercise such as we have identified with an asterisk* in the following series of routines. You will find that chest work will not affect your other exercises as much as shoulder and arm work. To fully benefit from your specialization, you should not attempt to carry the same work load on the individual body parts as with the chest workout.

Do the following routine of exercises for a period of six weeks, three days per week. Persons who have been exercising with weights for a period of time should bypass routine #1. You are the best judge of what routine is suitable for your particular training experience. It is our belief that anyone can use Programs 2, 3, 4, 5 and make outstanding gains, regardless of the length of time they have been working out.

Complete Movement

Make complete movements when exercising. A complete movement is full extension and contraction of the muscle being worked on. In chest work, effort should be made to stretch or extend the pectoral muscles. Bringing the arms across the chest or the hands together in front of the chest is a contraction. You must make a definite lockout of the elbows and force the dumbbells together when doing bent arm laterals and incline press or incline laterals and declines, etc.

Chest Development

When building a big chest, the first efforts should be directed toward increasing the rib box itself; then, strive for muscle development. Should one neglect to enlarge the rib cage, it will be extremely difficult to work the rib cage once the pectoral muscles have been developed. The strongest muscles

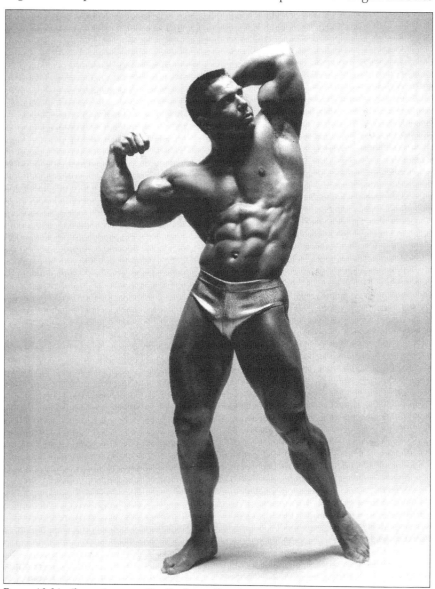

Even with his ribcage in repose Pearl's chest still maintains magnificent shape.

will do the work, unless extreme concentration is used, forcing the muscle you wish to work to do the work.

Breathing

A large impressive chest is an asset to anyone. Special effort should be taken in the beginning to enlarge the rib cage, as this houses your lungs, which are a very essential part of your body function. After a reasonable size is attained, the muscle may be worked to its maximum. Once the rib box is enlarged, it does not decrease in size like an unused muscle.

Distance runners and swimmers develop large chests through forced breathing. Bear in mind that this is not shallow breathing, but deep forced breathing. The majority of us do not place enough emphasis on deep breathing. It takes much effort to take a full breath and hold it, stressing a full usage of our lungs.

Therefore, we recommend that the person desiring a big well developed chest make a special effort to enlarge his rib box through forced and deep breathing. After a period of time is spent on this, then work hard to develop the muscles covering the rib box. The muscle will grow by exercising the chest, hut many people spend too much time and effort building big pectorals and give no thought to real chest expansion.

This page has been intentionally left blank.

Chapter 5

Equipment Needed

Equipment needed to perform the exercises in this training guide.

- Barbell
- Dumbbells
- Flat Bench
- Stool
- Incline Bench
- Block
- Parallel Bars

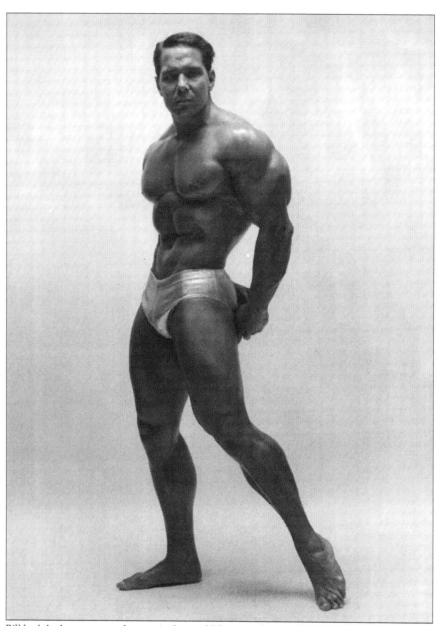

Bill had the largest muscular arm in the world for several years. It measured an honest cold 20 3/8 inches at a bodyweight of 218 pounds.

Chapter 6

Course One

EXERCISES:

1. Medium Grip Push-Ups on Floor	2 sets of 5-15
2. Bent Arm Lateral	2 sets of 8-10
3. Straight Arm Dumbbell Pullover	2 sets of 8-10
4. Medium Grip Barbell Bench Press	2 sets of 8-10

- Follow this course of exercises for a six week period
- Do Three Workouts per Week

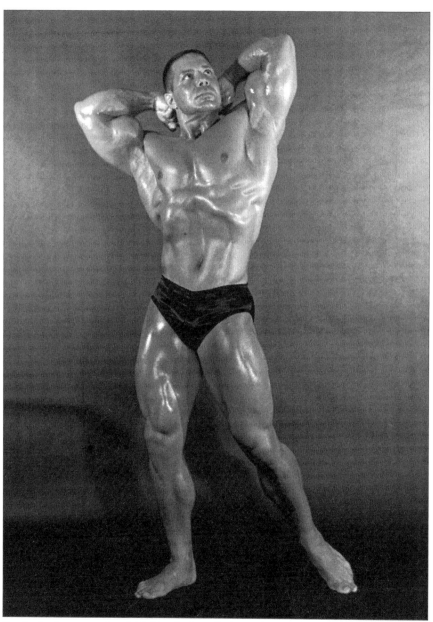

Pearl's chest was a weak point in his physique during early years. Hard work paid dividends.

MEDIUM GRIP PUSH-UPS ON FLOOR

Muscle Group: Pectorals and triceps
Degree of Difficulty: Intermediate
Start this exercise with the body in the position as shown in illustration #1. Your hands should be placed about twenty-four inches apart. Keep your body rigid and lower yourself to the position shown in illustration #2. Pause at the bottom and then push back to starting position. Inhale as you lower yourself and exhale while returning to starting position.

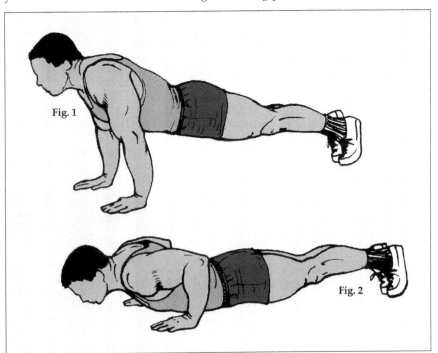

Fig. 1

Fig. 2

BENT ARM LATERAL

Muscle Group: Outer pectorals
Degree of Difficulty: Intermediate

Lie on a flat bench with the dumbbells together at arm's length above the shoulders The palms of the hands should be facing each other. Slowly lower the dumbbells to the down position so the dumbbells are approximately even with the chest but out about ten inches from each side of the chest. Notice that the elbows are drawn downwards and back so they are in line with the ears. The forearms are slightly out of a vertical position. The press back to starting position is done by using the same arc as in letting the dumbbells down. Inhale at the beginning of the exercise and exhale at the finish.

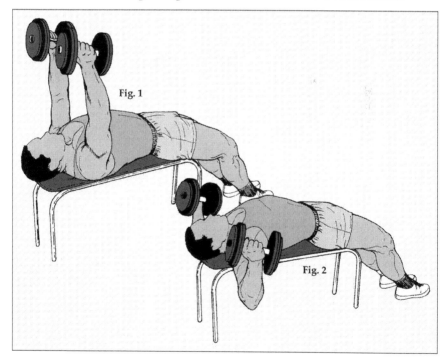

Fig. 1

Fig. 2

STRAIGHT ARM DUMBBELL PULLOVER

Muscle Group: Pectorals and rib cage
Degree of Difficulty: Intermediate

Lie supine on a flat bench with your head as close to the end of the bench as possible. Place your hands flat against the inside plate of a dumbbell. With the dumbbell held at arm's length above the chest, take a deep breath and lower the dumbbell in a semicircular motion over the chest and head to a position behind your head that brings no discomfort to the shoulder area. From this position, return the dumbbell to starting position, still keeping the elbows in a locked position. Exhale as you reach the starting position. Keep the head down, your chest held high, breathe heavily and do not raise your hips off the bench.

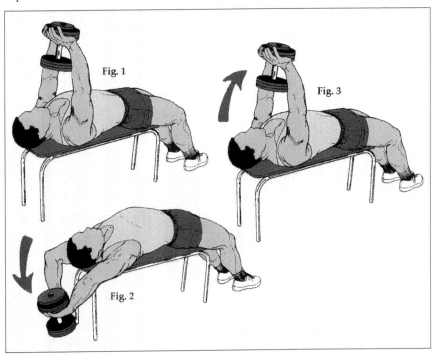

Fig. 1

Fig. 3

Fig. 2

MEDIUM GRIP BARBELL BENCH PRESS

Muscle Group: Outer pectorals
Degree of Difficulty: Intermediate

Lie in a supine position on a flat bench with your legs positioned at the sides of the bench and your feet flat on the floor. Using a hand grip that is about six inches wider than your shoulder width, bring the barbell to arm's length above the chest but in line with the shoulders. Lower the barbell to a position on the chest that is about an inch below the nipples of the pectorals. Note from the illustration that the elbows are back and the chest is held high. Inhale as the barbell is lowered to the chest and exhale as you push the barbell back to arm's length. Do not relax and drop the weight on the chest but lower it with complete control making a definite pause at the chest before pressing it back to starting position. Keep the head on the bench and do not arch the back too sharply as to raise your hips off the bench.

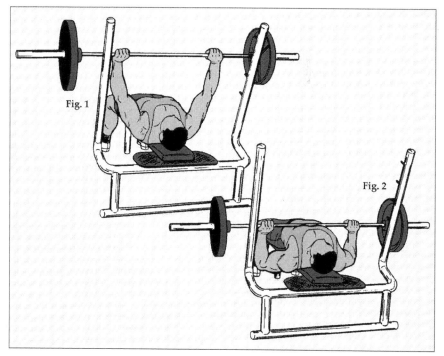

Chapter 7

Course Two

EXERCISES:

1. Incline Lateral	3 sets of 8-10
2. Bent Arm Barbell Pullover	3 sets of 8-10
3. Dips	3 sets of 8-10
4. Flat Dumbbell Fly	3 sets of 10

- Follow this course of exercises for a six week period
- Do Three Workouts per Week

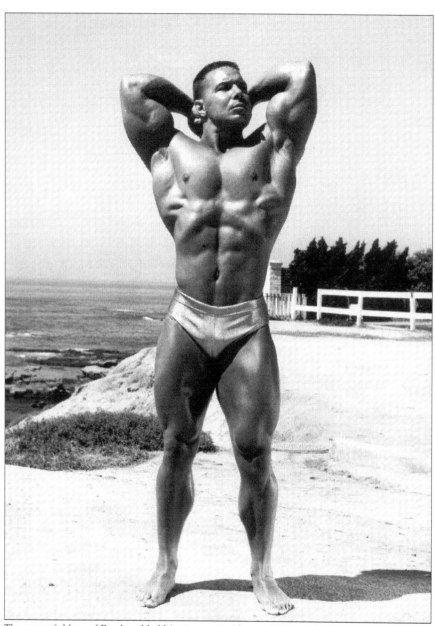

The powerful legs of Pearl enabled him to squat with over 600 pounds, something few men had done prior to 1960.

INCLINE LATERAL

Muscle Group: Upper pectorals
Degree of Difficulty: Intermediate

Use a hand position on the dumbbells similar to that of holding a barbell. Start with the dumbbells together at arm's length above the shoulders. Slowly lower them to the down position so the dumbbells are approximately even with the chest but about ten inches from each side of the chest. Notice that the elbows are drawn downwards and back so they are in line with the ears. The forearms are slightly out of a vertical position. The press back to starting position is done by using the same arc as in letting the dumbbells down. Inhale at the beginning of the exercise and exhale at the finish.

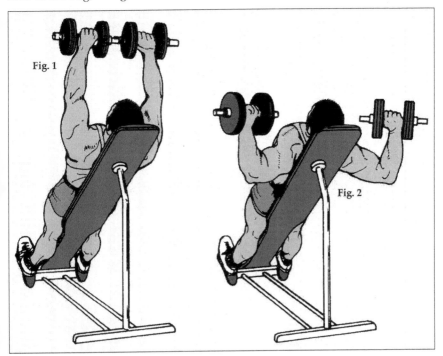

Fig. 1

Fig. 2

BENT ARM BARBELL PULLOVER

Muscle Group: Upper pectorals and rib cage
Degree of Difficulty: Intermediate

Lie supine on a flat bench with your shoulders at the end of the bench and your head pointing downward towards the floor. With a barbell on your chest resting in line with the nipples of the pectorals, use a hand grip that is about fourteen inches wide. Keeping the elbows in during the entire exercise, take a deep breath and lower the weight over your chest and face, keeping the barbell as close to the body as you can without scraping your nose. Continue to lower the weight until it touches the floor, or as low as is a comfortable position for you. Pull the barbell back to the chest, using the same path in which you lowered it. Exhale as you are doing so. Be sure to breathe heavily, keep the elbows in, and hold the chest high.

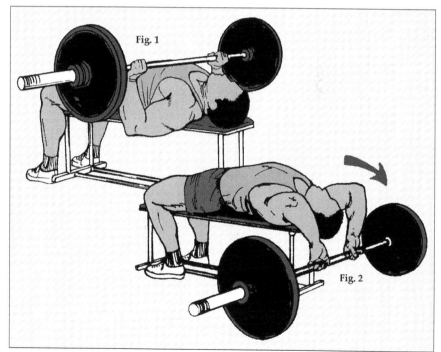

Fig. 1

Fig. 2

DIPS

Muscle Group: Pectorals and triceps
Degree of Difficulty: Difficult

Use a set of parallel bars or a regular dip stand for this exercise. Position yourself on the bars so you are held erect by your arms but able to drop to a low position without having your feet touch the floor. Keep your elbows into your sides as much as possible while lowering your body downward by bending your arms. You should continue downward until your forearms and biceps come together. Pause a short time and then press yourself back to arm's length forcing a lock out of the elbows thereby contracting the triceps and pectoral muscles. Do not let your body swing back and forth during this exercise. With a little practice and concentration, it will be very easy for you to control the body position. Inhale as you lower yourself and exhale as you push yourself back to starting position.

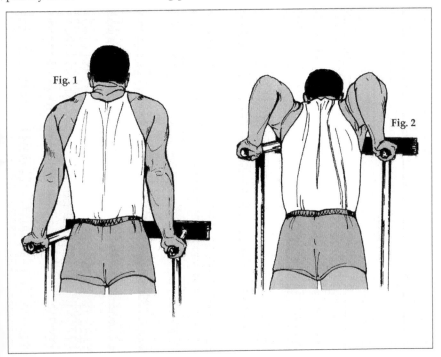

Fig. 1

Fig. 2

FLAT DUMBBELL FLY

Muscle Group: Outer pectorals
Degree of Difficulty: Intermediate

Lie supine on a flat bench with two light dumbbells at arm's length above the shoulders with the palms of the hands facing each other. Keeping the arms as straight as possible, lower the dumbbells out to each side of the chest in a semicircular motion until the weights are about even with the sides of your chest but back slightly so they are nearly in line with your ears. From this position return the weights back above the chest using the same path in which you used originally. Exhale as you reach the top position. You must breathe heavily, hold your chest high, keep your head on the bench and concentrate on the pectorals.

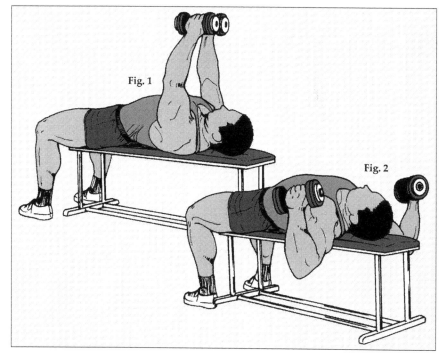

Fig. 1

Fig. 2

Chapter 8

Course Three

EXERCISES:

1. Medium Grip Barbell Bench Press	4 sets of 8
2. Straight Arm Dumbbell Pullover Across Bench	3 sets of 10-12
3. Bent Arm Dumbbell Pullover and Press	4 sets of 8
4. Lying Chest Cross Over	3 sets of 10

- Follow this course of exercises for a six week period
- Do Three Workouts per Week

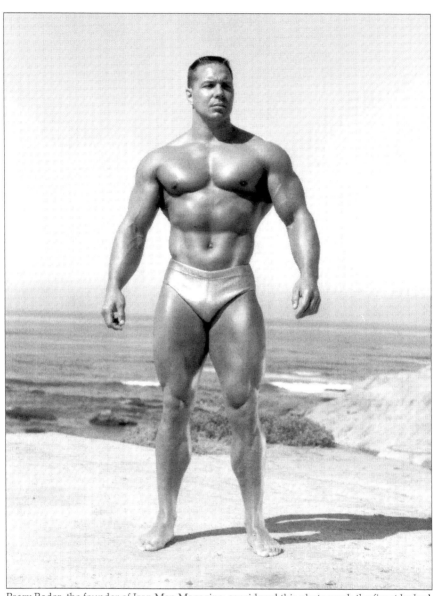

Peary Rader, the founder of Iron Man Magazine, considered this photograph the finest he had ever seen representing bodybuilding.

MEDIUM GRIP BARBELL BENCH PRESS

Muscle Group: Outer pectorals
Degree of Difficulty: Intermediate

Lie in a supine position on a flat bench with your legs positioned at the sides of the bench and your feet flat on the floor. Using a hand grip that is about six inches wider than your shoulder width, bring the barbell to arm's length above the chest but in line with the shoulders. Lower the barbell to a position on the chest that is about an inch below the nipples of the pectorals. Note from the illustration that the elbows are back and the chest is held high. Inhale as the barbell is lowered to the chest and exhale as you push the barbell back to arm's length. Do not relax and drop the weight on the chest but lower it with complete control making a definite pause at the chest before pressing it back to starting position. Keep the head on the bench and do not arch the back too sharply as to raise your hips off the bench.

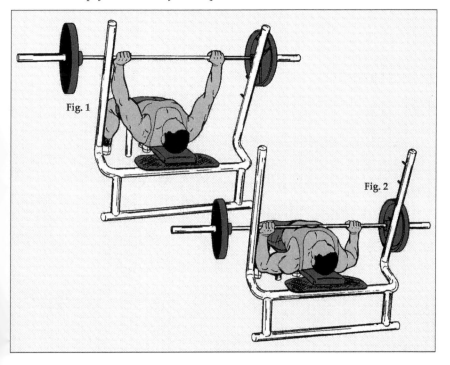

STRAIGHT ARM DUMBBELL PULLOVER ACROSS BENCH

Muscle Group: Pectorals and rib cage
Degree of Difficulty: Intermediate

Lie supine across a bench with your upper back supporting the weight of your upper body and your head off the bench hanging in a downward position. Keep your body and legs nearly straight while trying to drop the hips downward slightly to help raise the rib cage. Place your hands flat against the inside plate of a dumbbell. With the dumbbell held at arm's length above the chest, take a deep breath and lower the weight in a semicircular movement over and behind your head until it is lowered as far back as possible without bringing discomfort to the shoulder area. From this low position, return the dumbbell to starting position, still keeping the elbows in a locked position. Exhale as you reach the top. Keep the head in a downward position, breathe heavily and do not raise the hips.

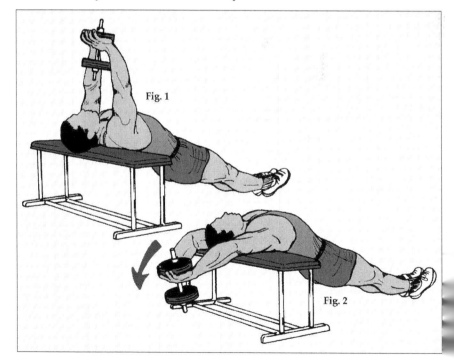

Fig. 1

Fig. 2

BENT ARM DUMBBELL PULLOVER AND PRESS

Muscle Group: Pectorals and rib cage
Degree of Difficulty: Difficult

Lie supine on a flat bench with your shoulders at the end of the bench and your head pointing downward towards the floor. With a dumbbell in each hand, place the weights to the sides of your chest about even with the nipples of the pectorals. Keeping the elbows in during the entire exercise, take a deep breath and lower the weights over and past your face so they just pass by your ears on their way downwards towards the floor. Continue to lower the dumbbells until they reach the floor, or go as low as possible without bringing discomfort to the shoulder area. Then pull the dumbbells back to the position at the sides of the chest using the same path in which you lowered them. Then press the dumbbells to arm's length above the chest, keeping the palms of the hands facing each other. As you lower the weights, let your air out. Both movements constitute one repetition. Be sure to breathe heavily, keep the elbows in, and hold the rib cage high.

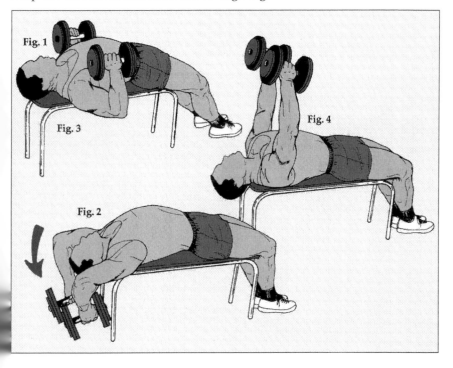

LYING CHEST CROSS OVER

Muscle Group: Outer and inner pectorals
Degree of Difficulty: Intermediate

Lie on a flat bench with two light dumbbells at arm's length above the shoulders. Keeping the arms as straight as possible, lower the dumbbells out to each side of the chest in a semicircular motion until the weights are about even with the sides of your chest. As you bring the dumbbells back to starting position over the chest, turn the dumbbells so the palms of the hands are facing away from your head and cross your arms over your chest, trying to cramp the pectoral muscles. Bend your elbows slightly so you can force your arms across the body more and tighten the pectorals. Alternate the crossing of the arms with each repetition you perform. Inhale as you lower the dumbbells and exhale as you cross your arms.

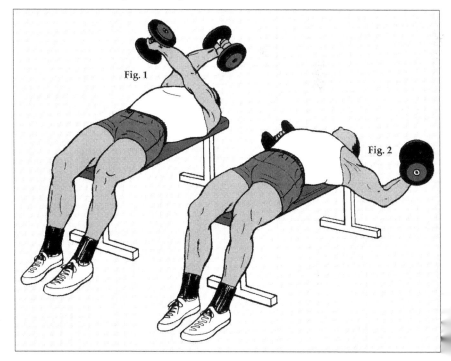

Fig. 1

Fig. 2

Chapter 9

Course Four

EXERCISES:

1. Wide Grip Incline Barbell Bench Press	4 sets of 8
2. Decline Dumbbell Fly	4 sets of 8
3. Bent Arm Barbell Pullover and Press	3 sets of 8
4. Straight Arm Dumbbell Pullover	3 sets of 10
5. Decline Around the World	3 sets of 10-20

- Follow this course of exercises for a six week period
- Do Three Workouts per Week

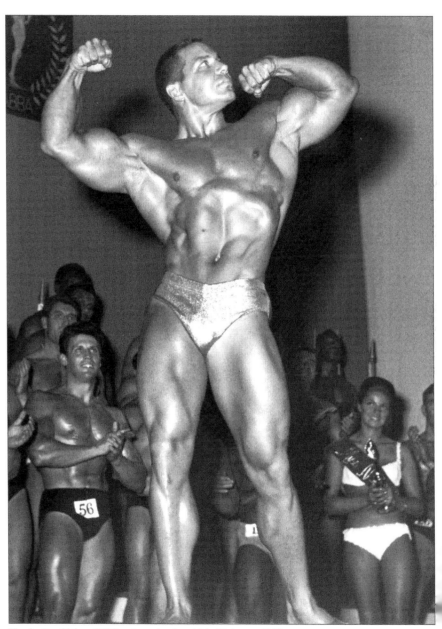

The fruits of labor. Bill Pearl, professional Mr. Universe 1967.

WIDE GRIP INCLINE BARBELL BENCH PRESS

Muscle Group: Outer and upper pectorals
Degree of Difficulty: Difficult

Lie back on an incline bench. Using a collar to collar grip, lower the barbell from arm's length above the shoulders to a position on the chest that is about three inches above the nipples of the pectorals. Note from the illustrations that the elbows are back and the forearms are nearly vertical as the weight is lowered. Inhale as you lower the barbell and exhale as you press it back to starting position. Do not relax as you press it back to starting position. Do not drop the barbell on the upper chest but lower it in a controlled manner, making a definite pause at the upper chest before pressing it back to arm's length. Keep your head on the bench and hold the chest high but do not raise the hips off the bench.

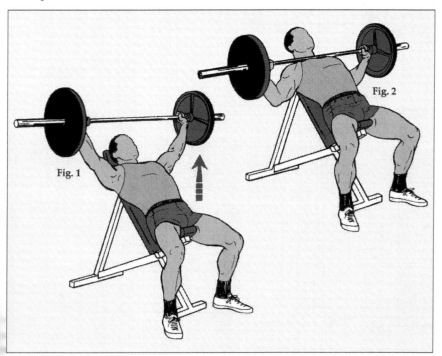

Fig. 1

Fig. 2

DECLINE DUMBBELL FLY

Muscle Group: Lower pectorals
Degree of Difficulty: Intermediate

Lie on a decline bench with two light dumbbells at arm's length above the shoulders with the palms of the hands facing each other. Keeping the arms as straight as possible, lower the dumbbells out to each side of the chest but slightly back so they are nearly in line with your ears. From this position return the weights back above the chest using the same path in which you used originally. Exhale as you reach the top position. You must breathe heavily, hold your chest high, keep your head on the bench and concentrate on the pectorals.

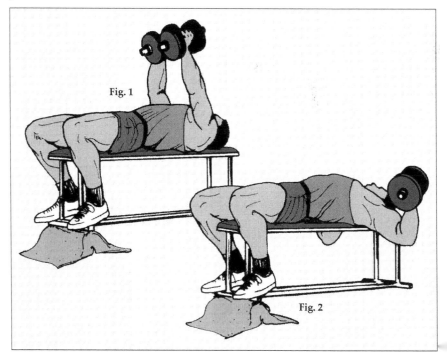

Fig. 1

Fig. 2

BENT ARM BARBELL PULLOVER AND PRESS

Muscle Group: Pectorals and rib cage
Degree of Difficulty: Difficult

Lie supine on a flat bench with your shoulders at the end of the bench and your head pointing downward towards the floor, with a barbell on your chest resting in line with the nipples of the pectorals using a hand grip that is about fourteen inches wide. Keeping the elbows in during the entire exercise, take a deep breath and lower the barbell over your chest and face keeping the weight as close to the body and face as you can without scraping your nose. Continue to lower the weight until it touches the floor or as low as is a comfortable position for your shoulders, pull the barbell back to the chest using the same path in which you lowered it. Then press the barbell to arm's length above the chest and as you are lowering the weight let your air out. Both movements will constitute one repetition. Be sure to breathe heavily, keep the elbows in and hold the rib cage high.

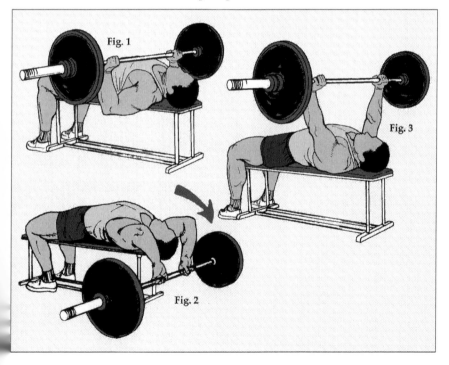

Fig. 1

Fig. 2

Fig. 3

STRAIGHT ARM DUMBBELL PULLOVER

Muscle Group: Pectorals and rib cage
Degree of Difficulty: Intermediate

Lie supine on a flat bench with your head as close to the end of the bench as possible. Place your hands flat against the inside plate of a dumbbell. With the dumbbell held at arm's length above the chest, take a deep breath and lower the dumbbell in a semicircular motion over the chest and head to a position behind your head that brings no discomfort to the shoulder area. From this position, return the dumbbell to starting position, still keeping the elbows in a locked position. Exhale as you reach the starting position. Keep the head down, your chest held high, breathe heavily and do not raise your hips off the bench.

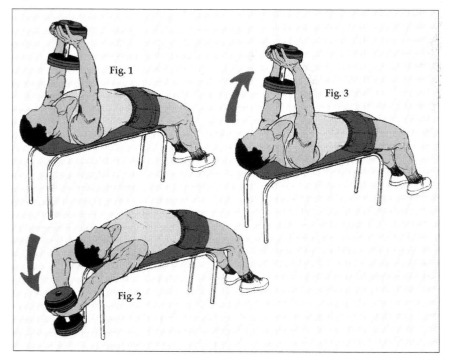

DECLINE AROUND THE WORLD

Muscle Group: Lower pectorals
Degree of Difficulty: Intermediate

Lie on a decline bench with a dumbbell held in each hand, having the palms of your hands facing each other while the dumbbells are held on each thigh just below the groin area. Keep the elbows slightly bent but have them locked out while bringing the weights out and around in a circular motion to the sides of the body past the waist, chest and head until the dumbbells come together behind your head at arm's length. As you are bringing the dumbbells to the position behind your head you should turn your wrists so the palms will be facing upward at the half way position of the exercise. Return the dumbbells in the same path in which you brought them behind your head. Inhale as you commence the exercise and exhale as you bring the weights back to the top of the thighs.

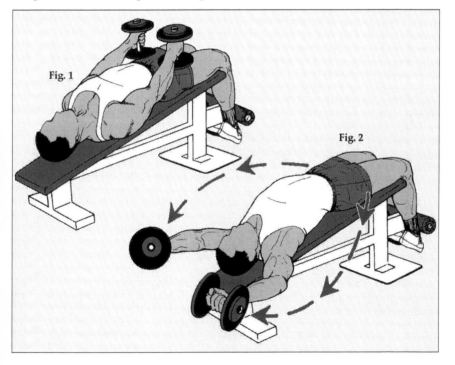

Fig. 1

Fig. 2

This page has been intentionally left blank.

Chapter 10

Course Five

EXERCISES:

1. Bent Arm Lateral	2 sets of 10
2. Medium Grip Push-Ups on Floor	3 sets of 10-15
3. Pec Cross Over on High Pulley	3 sets of 8-10
4. Incline Compound	4 sets of 6-8
5. Dips	4 sets of 6-8
6. Decline Around the World	2 sets of 12

- Follow this course of exercises for a six week period
- Do Three Workouts per Week

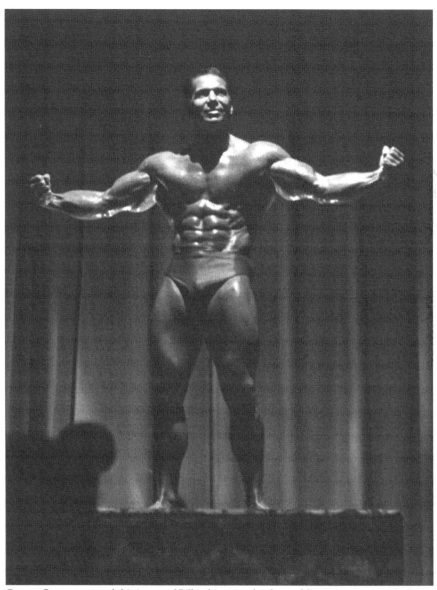

George Coates captured this image of Bill in his second to last public posing appearance in the United States before going to London to win the 1971 Mr. Universe title. Shape, size, and depth in abundance.

BENT ARM LATERAL

Muscle Group: Outer pectorals
Degree of Difficulty: Intermediate

Lie on a flat bench with the dumbbells together at arm's length above the shoulders The palms of the hands should be facing each other. Slowly lower the dumbbells to the down position so the dumbbells are approximately even with the chest but out about ten inches from each side of the chest. Notice that the elbows are drawn downwards and back so they are in line with the ears. The forearms are slightly out of a vertical position. The press back to starting position is done by using the same arc as in letting the dumbbells down. Inhale at the beginning of the exercise and exhale at the finish.

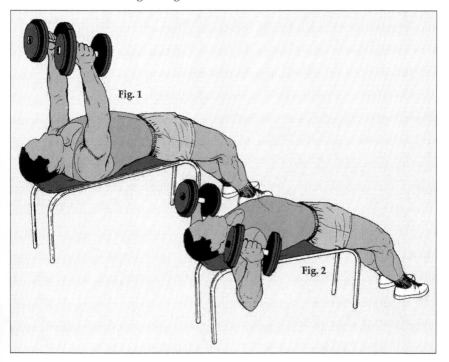

Fig. 1

Fig. 2

MEDIUM GRIP PUSH-UPS ON FLOOR

Muscle Group: Pectorals and triceps
Degree of Difficulty: Intermediate

Start this exercise with the body in the position as shown in illustration #1. Your hands should be placed about twenty-four inches apart. Keep your body rigid and lower yourself to the position shown in illustration #2. Pause at the bottom and then push back to starting position. Inhale as you lower yourself and exhale while returning to starting position.

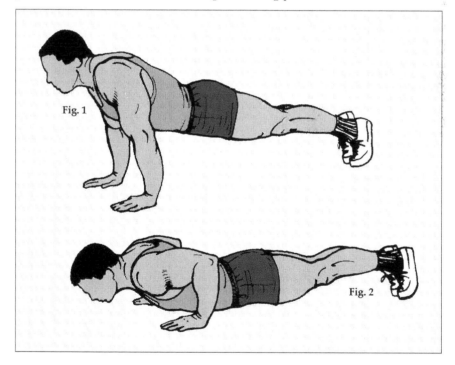

Fig. 1

Fig. 2

PEC CROSS OVER ON HIGH PULLEY

Muscle Group: Upper and inner pectorals
Degree of Difficulty: Intermediate

Use wall pulley that has handles at the top. Stand so your side is facing the pulley. Grasp the top handle and step out away from the pulley so your arm is totally extended and there is tension on the cable of the wall pulley. From this position, keep your arm straight, pull your arm across your chest not letting the hand drop any lower than the height of your shoulder. The thumb of the hand should be facing up during the exercise. As you are pulling the cable across your chest, concentrate on the inner portion of the pectoral trying to get it to do the majority of the work. Inhale as you commence the pull and exhale as you let the cable back to starting position. Complete the prescribed number of repetitions with one arm and then change to the other side and complete the prescribed number of repetitions with that arm.

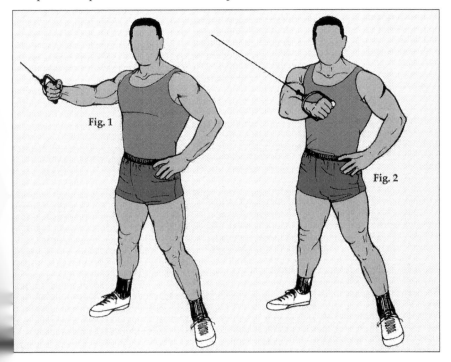

INCLINE COMPOUND

Muscle Group: Upper pectorals
Degree of Difficulty: Difficult

This is a two-motion exercise so care should be used in following the directions and studying the illustration. Lie on an incline bench with two dumbbells at arm's length overhead. With the palms facing out, lower the dumbbells in a half circle motion, keeping the elbows back in line with the ears as the weights are lowered. Lower the dumbbells until they are approximately even with the chest but out about ten inches from each side of the chest. From this position press the dumbbells back to starting position still keeping the elbows back in line with the ears. When you have reached the top position, change the position of the dumbbells by turning your hands so the palms are now facing each other. From this position lower the dumbbells straight down to the sides of the chest. Keeping the elbows in close to the sides as the weights are lowered. Bring the dumbbells back to starting position. This will constitute a single repetition. Change hand positions and start the exercise again. Inhale at the top and exhale at the top of each movement.

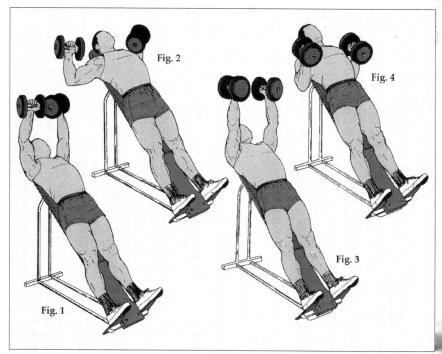

Fig. 1 Fig. 2 Fig. 3 Fig. 4

DIPS

Muscle Group: Pectorals and triceps
Degree of Difficulty: Difficult

Use a set of parallel bars or a regular dip stand for this exercise. Position yourself on the bars so you are held erect by your arms but able to drop to a low position without having your feet touch the floor. Keep your elbows into your sides as much as possible while lowering your body downward by bending your arms. You should continue downward until your forearms and biceps come together. Pause a short time and then press yourself back to arm's length forcing a lock out of the elbows thereby contracting the triceps and pectoral muscles. Do not let your body swing back and forth during this exercise. With a little practice and concentration, it will be very easy for you to control the body position. Inhale as you lower yourself and exhale as you push yourself back to starting position.

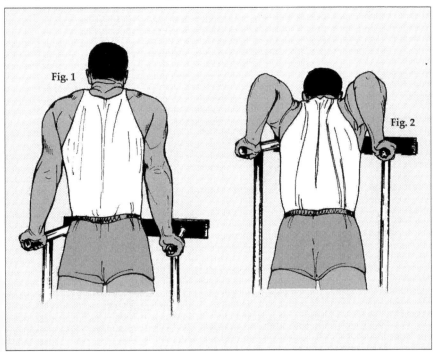

DECLINE AROUND THE WORLD

Muscle Group: Lower pectorals
Degree of Difficulty: Intermediate

Lie on a decline bench with a dumbbell held in each hand, having the palms of your hands facing each other while the dumbbells are held on each thigh just below the groin area. Keep the elbows slightly bent but have them locked out while bringing the weights out and around in a circular motion to the sides of the body past the waist, chest and head until the dumbbells come together behind your head at arm's length. As you are bringing the dumbbells to the position behind your head you should turn your wrists so the palms will be facing upward at the half way position of the exercise. Return the dumbbells in the same path in which you brought them behind your head. Inhale as you commence the exercise and exhale as you bring the weights back to the top of the thighs.

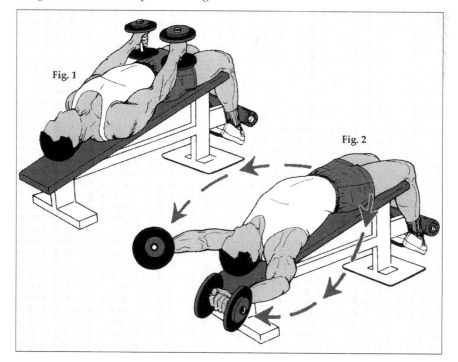

Chapter 11

Training Comments

It is our belief that the bench press is over-rated as a chest developing exercise. Some men, who have developed their chest outstandingly, claim the bench press is their main exercise. Our experience, both personally and training others, is that there are many exercises more effective in building large well shaped pectorals.

Bench pressing is a great asset in increasing one's power. It helps to build a large chest through the growth stimuli. As far as pectorals are concerned, the most effective are the bent arm laterals, chest crossovers, incline press, declines and flying motion.

Hints

It is important to place stress on the pectorals and not use the strength of the triceps when doing forced lockouts in incline press, bent arm laterals, straight arm pullover, declines and exercises of that nature.

Deep breathing is very important when exercising, for it gives your system much more oxygen with which to work and helps you gain in chest expansion.

When building the upper pectorals with exercises such as incline press with both barbells and dumbbells, you must stretch the muscles when lowering dumbbells to down position and force dumbbells together at top position to get a full extension and contraction.

Keeping elbows back toward top of head and forearms vertical, works the muscle much more than when allowing dumbbells to come in toward the sides.

Posture

Posture is very important. No matter how hard you work to build your chest, both structure and muscle wise, if you slouch, slump or round the shoulders, your work will be in vain. Stand erect with head high and back straight. This will improve your appearance as much as adding three or four inches in diameter to your chest

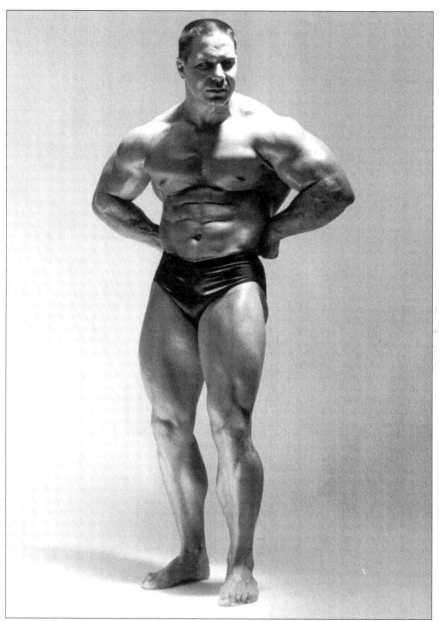

Pearl's calf measurement was 19 1/4 inches at the time of this photograph. Because of his excellent symmetry, this huge size does not seem out of place.

This page has been intentionally left blank.

83586482R00031

Made in the USA
San Bernardino, CA
27 July 2018